ILEOSTOMY DIET FOR NEWLY DIAGNOSED

Complete Six Weeks Post-Surgery Recipes, Meal Plans, Expert Tips, And Lifestyle Recommendations To Combat Ileostomy And Thrive After Surgery

DR. ERIC TRISTAN

CONTENTS

DISCLAIMER

The information provided in this book, is intended for informational purposes only. The content is not intended to be a substitute for professional medical advice, diagnosis, or treatment. Always seek the advice of your physician or other qualified health provider with any questions you may have regarding a medical condition. Never disregard professional medical advice or delay in seeking it because of something you have read in this book.

The author of this book has made reasonable efforts to ensure that the information provided is accurate and up-to-date at the time of publication. However, the author makes no representations or warranties of any kind, express or implied, about the completeness, accuracy, reliability, suitability, or availability of the information contained within these pages.

Any reliance you place on the information provided in this book is strictly at your own risk. The author shall not be liable for any loss, injury, or damage arising from the use of this book or the information contained herein.

The mention or reference to any individuals, products, websites, organizations, or other names within this book does not imply endorsement by the author. The inclusion of such references is solely for informational purposes and does not constitute an endorsement or recommendation.

Furthermore, the author disclaims any association or affiliation with any individuals, products, websites, organizations, or other names mentioned in this book.

It is important to consult with a qualified healthcare professional before making any dietary or lifestyle changes, especially if you have a medical condition. Each individual's health situation is unique, and what works for one person may not work for another.

Again, the information provided in this book is not intended to diagnose, treat, cure, or prevent any disease or health condition. Always seek the advice of a physician or other qualified health provider regarding any medical questions or concerns you may have.

Thank you for your understanding and for taking the necessary precautions when considering the information presented in this book.

ABOUT THIS BOOK

This book publication entitled "Ileostomy Diet" provides comprehensive information on an essential element of post-operative care for patients undergoing ileostomy procedures. This book provides an extensive assortment of subjects, including emotional support, dietary guidelines, and caregiver education. As a result, it is an indispensable resource for fans, patients, and healthcare practitioners.

This book commences with a comprehensive introduction to ileostomy, elucidating the objectives and classifications of this surgical procedure for the benefit of the readership. Patients must possess a comprehensive understanding of the underlying reasoning behind ileostomy to successfully adjust to their newly prescribed dietary needs.

An aspect of merit that this book possesses is its prioritization of preparation and incremental adaptation to dietary modifications. Through the provision of dietary guidelines both before and following ileostomy surgery, readers are furnished with the information and resources essential for effectively managing the complexities of an ileostomy diet.

The comprehensive analysis encompassing essential nutrients and electrolyte monitoring, guidance on hydration, fiber consumption management, and avoidance and inclusion of foods provides pragmatic perspectives on sustaining optimal nutritional status and general health. This book reaffirms its dedication to catering to the varied requirements of patients by taking into account specific demographics, including expectant women with ileostomy and infants.

Furthermore, this book explores the psychological and affective dimensions of dietary modifications, acknowledging the significant influence that such changes can exert on the quality of life of an individual. Through the provision of coping mechanisms for digestive challenges and recommendations for pursuing professional dietary guidance, this book enables readers to proactively manage their health and successfully acclimate to their newly adopted dietary regimen.

This practical guidebook's utility is further enhanced by the incorporation of personalized ileostomy diet plans, prevalent challenges, and long-term maintenance recommendations, which offer guidance to individuals navigating life with an ileostomy. In its entirety, "Ileostomy Diet" serves as a valuable resource, offering thorough assistance and direction to individuals initiating the process of managing their diet after undergoing surgery.

CHAPTER ONE

An Overview Of Ileostomy

Surgically, an ileostomy is performed by creating a fistula, or incision in the abdominal wall, through which the ileum, a portion of the small intestine, is taken to the skin's surface.

When a portion of the colon or rectum must be excised or bypassed as a result of disease, injury, or other medical conditions, this surgical procedure is usual. When the body's natural digestive pathway is compromised, an alternative pathway for waste material to be expelled is established through the construction of an ileostomy.

Ileostomy surgery can be performed on individuals for a multitude of reasons. These reasons may include inflammatory bowel diseases such as Crohn's disease or ulcerative colitis, colorectal malignancy, gastrointestinal tract congenital abnormalities, or trauma.

A person's daily living may be substantially altered by the insertion of an ileostomy, necessitating modifications to one's diet, way of life, and self-care regimen.

Stoma: A pouching system adhered to the skin accumulates feces and intestinal fluids as they depart the body through the stoma, which resembles a tiny, pinkish-red opening on the abdomen. Individual differences in stool output frequency and consistency may result from dietary and hydration patterns, as well as the degree of intestinal resection performed during surgery.

Frequently, adjusting to life with an ileostomy necessitates mastery of effective stoma and associated appliance management skills. By receiving appropriate education, support, and resources, individuals can successfully navigate the challenges associated with having an ileostomy and still lead satisfying lives.

Types And Objectives Of Ileostomy

By diverting intestinal contents away from a diseased or malfunctioning segment of the gastrointestinal tract, an ileostomy serves as its primary function. Ileostomy surgery assists patients with a variety of gastrointestinal conditions in managing complications, alleviating symptoms, and enhancing their overall quality of life through the establishment of an alternative pathway for waste elimination.

An assortment of ileostomy types exist, each possessing distinct attributes and indications:

1. Extremity Ileostomy: To create the stoma, this variety of ileostomy requires bringing the extremity of the ileum through the abdominal wall. End ileostomies are frequently conducted when the entire colon and rectum are removed to treat familial adenomatous polyposis (FAP), colorectal malignancy, or ulcerative colitis.

2. Loop Ileostomy: To produce the stoma during a loop ileostomy, a segment of the ileum is introduced to the abdominal surface. In contrast to an end ileostomy, intestinal contents are temporarily diverted during a loop ileostomy. It is frequently designed to rest and secure a section of the colon or rectum in the aftermath of an operation, inflammation, or trauma. Reversal of loop ileostomies is possible when the underlying condition resolves or improves.

3. Continent ileostomy, also known as cock pouch ileostomy, differs from conventional ileostomies in that an internal reservoir or pouch is created from a segment of the ileum. The pouch incorporates a valve mechanism that regulates the discharge of feces, enabling individuals to handle waste removal without the need for an external pouching system. Constant ileostomies necessitate vigilant self-catheterization to routinely defecate the pouch.

The recommended ileostomy type is determined by the surgical considerations, the underlying condition, and the patient's medical requirements and preferences.

A variety of healthcare practitioners—dietitians, enterostomal therapists, and surgeons—are essential in the assessment, coordination, and administration of the care provided to patients undergoing ileostomy surgery.

Preparation For A Dietary Ileostomy

In addition to physical adjustments, dietary modifications are required to regulate stool consistency, prevent dehydration, and preserve optimal nutrition when adjusting to life with an ileostomy.

The establishment of an ileostomy diet necessitates the cooperation of registered dietitians, healthcare providers, and patients to accommodate specific dietary requirements and preferences.

Essential considerations for preparing a diet for an ileostomy are as follows:

1. Gradual Transition: Individuals who have undergone ileostomy surgery may encounter alterations in their bowel function and digestion. It is imperative to incrementally incorporate dietary modifications while closely monitoring the impact of various foods on gas production, stool output, and overall comfort.

2. It is of the utmost importance that individuals with an ileostomy maintain adequate hydration, as increased fluid loss may result from a greater discharge of liquid excrement. Consisting of electrolyte-rich beverages and copious amounts of water consumed throughout the day aid in the prevention of dehydration and electrolyte imbalances.

3. The consumption of fiber, although crucial for maintaining digestive health, can cause an increase in defecation frequency and volume, which may

pose challenges for individuals who have an ileostomy. By incorporating soluble fibers derived from whole cereals, fruits, and vegetables into one's diet gradually, digestive movements can be better regulated without an increase in stool output.

4. A limited residue diet restricts the intake of foods that are particularly rich in indigestible material, roughage, and fiber. This can facilitate the passage of stool through the stoma and reduce the likelihood of obstructions or irritation by decreasing stool frequency and bulk.

5. Maintaining a balanced and nutrient-dense diet is crucial for individuals with an ileostomy, notwithstanding any dietary restrictions they may have. A balanced diet that includes foods from various food groups promotes sufficient consumption of vital nutrients, vitamins, minerals, and protein, which are all essential for proper functioning, energy generation, and overall health.

Through close collaboration with healthcare professionals and the implementation of suitable dietary strategies, individuals can optimize their nutritional status, digestive health, and postoperative quality of life while effectively managing their ileostomy diet. Constant monitoring, education, and support are essential elements of effective dietary management for individuals who have undergone ileostomy.

CHAPTER TWO

Dietary Guidelines Following Surgery

After undergoing ileostomy surgery, patients experience substantial alterations in their digestive system, which underscores the importance of adhering to dietary recommendations to facilitate recovery, avert complications, and enhance overall well-being. To facilitate waste elimination, an ileostomy entails redirecting a segment of the small intestine via an incision in the abdominal wall, thereby establishing a stoma. The following are crucial dietary recommendations for individuals who have undergone ileostomy surgery:

1. Commence using clear liquids:

Commence consuming clear liquids such as water, broth, clear fruit beverages, and herbal tea following surgery. These aid in the preservation of hydration and supply vital electrolytes while avoiding undue strain on the digestive system.

2. Develop Gradually:

Reintroduce solid foods to the diet gradually, beginning with mild, low-fiber alternatives. Reintroduce foods gradually while observing the effects on digestion and stool consistency.

3. Thoroughly chew:

A comprehensive chewing motion facilitates digestion and reduces the likelihood of blockages. Food particles are broken down by proper mastic, which facilitates digestion and absorption.

4. Observe Fiber Consumption:

At the outset, restrict the consumption of high-fiber foods like fresh fruits and vegetables, whole cereals, nuts, and seeds. Potential dehydration may result from the distress and increased stool output caused by high-fiber diets.

5. Remain Hydrated:

Individuals with an ileostomy need to maintain adequate hydration to prevent dehydration caused by increased fluid loss through the stoma. Consume copious amounts of fluids, including electrolyte solutions, herbal tea, and water, throughout the day.

6. Regulation of Gas-Generating Foods:

Consume foods in moderation that induce flatulence, including legumes, cabbage, broccoli, scallions, and carbonated beverages. Bloating and discomfort brought on by gas can exacerbate postoperative discomfort.

7. Avoid Foods That Cause Issues:

Avoid consuming foods that have the potential to obstruct or irritate the area surrounding the stoma, including fibrous vegetables such as celery and maize, difficult meats, popcorn, and almonds.

8. Observed Output:

Track the frequency, consistency, and production of bowel movements. Variations in bowel movements may serve as an indicator of dietary concerns or possible complications necessitating medical intervention.

9. Vitamin and dietary supplementation:

Consider integrating nutritional supplements or vitamins into one's diet, contingent upon specific dietary requirements, to promote general well-being and avert deficiencies.

10. Advice from a Dietitian:

Collaborate closely with a registered dietitian who possesses extensive experience in the management of diets for individuals undergoing ileostomy. In addition to addressing concerns, a dietitian can offer individualized dietary recommendations and assist in optimizing nutritional intake.

Foods That Are Introduced Gradually.

For individuals assimilating to life with an ileostomy, the incremental reintroduction of nutrients is vital. Postoperatively, the digestive system experiences substantial alterations, necessitating a period of adjustment to novel dietary regimens and food items. The following strategy is recommended for the incremental introduction of foods:

Phase One: Liquid Clarification

Immediately after surgery, begin with clear liquids such as water, bouillon, and herbal tea. Clear liquids aid in preventing dehydration and are easy on the digestive system.

Phase 2: Foods Low in Fibre

Incorporate foods that are low in fiber, including skinless potatoes, white bread, white rice, and pasta. These foods are less likely to induce discomfort or irritation and are easily digestible.

Phase Three: Vegetables and Fruits Preheated

Incorporate prepared fruits and vegetables into the diet gradually, as they are more easily digestible and milder in texture than their raw counterparts. Seeds, husks, and stiff fibers should be eliminated to reduce digestive issues.

Fourth Phase: Lean Proteins

Include in your diet lean proteins such as fish, skinless poultry, tofu, and eggs. By selecting poultry and meat that is tender, one can minimize the likelihood of experiencing digestive discomfort.

Phase 5: Foods Rich in Fibre (Optional)

Once the digestive system has returned to normal, incorporate high-fiber foods into the diet, including whole grains, legumes, and fibrous vegetables. To prevent complications, monitor tolerance and adjust fiber intake accordingly.

Phase 6: Dietary Individualization

Reintroduce customized foods gradually, taking into consideration individual preferences, intolerances, and nutritional requirements. Maintain a food journal to monitor reactions to various foods and detect possible intolerances or triggers.

Incorporating Foods Into An Ileostomy Diet

The primary objectives of an ileostomy diet are to ensure proper nutrition, prevent complications, and promote digestive health. The following are acceptable ingredients for an ileostomy diet:

1. Reduced-Fiber Foods:

Select refined cereals, white bread, white rice, and pasta as low-fiber alternatives. These foods are less likely to induce obstructions or irritation in the digestive tract.

2. Precooked Vegetables and Fruits:

Select prepared, mushy vegetables and fruits, including pureed potatoes, applesauce, mangoes, and steamed carrots. Fruits and vegetables are simpler to metabolize and the risk of digestive distress is diminished when they are cooked.

3. Lean protein sources include:

Incorporate well-prepared lean meats, skinless poultry, fish, eggs, tofu, and lean fish into your diet. Protein is particularly vital for tissue regeneration and general well-being, particularly in the period following surgical treatment.

4. Dairy Products, including:

Include in one's dietary intake dairy products such as yogurt, cheese, and lactose-free milk. Protein and calcium, both of which are vital for bone health and overall nutrition, are found in dairy products.

5. High-Nutrient Foods:

In moderation, incorporate nutrient-dense foods into your diet, such as avocados, almonds, seeds, and nut butter. These dietary items are rich in vital minerals, vitamins, and essential lipids that promote general health and wellness.

6. Sufficient hydration:

Consume copious amounts of fluids on an ongoing basis to prevent dehydration and ensure adequate hydration. For adequate hydration, water, herbal tea, electrolyte solutions, and clear fruit juices are all excellent options.

7. Supplementary Materials:

It is advisable to contemplate the use of dietary supplements or vitamins to mitigate the risk of potential nutrient deficiencies, especially in cases where specific foods are restricted or cause intolerance.

8. Well-Rested Meals:

To ensure proper nutrition and promote overall health, strive to incorporate a diverse range of foods from various food groups into well-balanced meals.

In summary, it is critical for individuals recovering from ileostomy surgery to adhere to a balanced ileostomy diet comprising a diverse selection of nutrient-dense foods, reintegrate foods gradually, and closely monitor their dietary tolerance. By adhering to these dietary recommendations and collaborating closely with healthcare practitioners, individuals can enhance their nutritional consumption, facilitate recovery, and elevate their overall quality of life.

CHAPTER THREE

Importance Of Hydration For Ileostomy Patients

It is imperative to maintain adequate hydration for all individuals, but it is especially critical for those who have undergone an ileostomy, which is a surgical procedure involving the creation of an orifice in the abdomen for waste passage following the removal of the colon and rectum, in whole or in part. Water absorption in the digestive tract is altered when an ileostomy is present; if not effectively managed, this can result in dehydration. Consequently, the health and well-being of ileostomy patients must consume an adequate amount of water.

1. Patients with an ileostomy should strive to ingest ample fluids daily to counterbalance the heightened susceptibility to dehydration. Although water is the optimal hydration medium, herbal infusions, clear broths, and electrolyte solutions may also provide additional benefits. Aim for a minimum of eight to

ten glasses of fluids daily, but feel free to modify as necessary, particularly in the presence of high temperatures or physical exertion.

2. It is critical that ileostomy patients routinely observe the discharge of their stoma. Variations in the consistency or volume of discharge may serve as an indicator of changes in hydration levels. A thicker or less frequent output may be indicative of dehydration, whereas a watery output may suggest overhydration. Patients and healthcare providers can identify trends and make necessary adjustments to fluid intake by maintaining a record of stoma discharge.

3. Electrolyte Replacement: Elevated ileostomy output can accelerate the loss of electrolytes including sodium, potassium, and magnesium. It is essential to replenish these electrolytes to preserve adequate hydration and avert imbalances. Electrolyte-dense foods such as potatoes, bananas, yogurt, and coconut water can aid in the natural replenishment of electrolytes lost.

4. Avoid Dehydrating Substances: Certain substances can worsen dehydration in patients who have undergone ileostomy. For instance, the diuretic properties of caffeine and alcohol can stimulate urine output and contribute to fluid depletion. By limiting or avoiding these beverages, dehydration can be avoided and hydration balance can be maintained.

5. Incorporate Hydrating Foods: In addition to fluids, ileostomy patients can benefit from hydration efforts supported by the consumption of hydrating foods. Veggies and fruits that are rich in water, including strawberries, watermelon, cucumbers, and citrus, can aid in the maintenance of a healthy body fluid level and supply vital vitamins and minerals.

6. It is advisable to seek guidance from a dietitian regarding hydration requirements, as they can differ among individuals due to factors such as age, weight, level of physical activity, and overall health condition. Ileostomy patients can benefit from the guidance of a registered dietitian specializing in gastrointestinal health when it comes to formulating

individualized hydration plans that are customized to their particular requirements and preferences.

In conclusion, ileostomy patients must ensure adequate hydration to promote their overall health and well-being. Individuals with an ileostomy can optimize their hydration status and reduce the likelihood of complications associated with dehydration by supplementing electrolytes, increasing fluid consumption, monitoring stoma output, refraining from dehydrating substances, incorporating hydrating foods, and consulting healthcare professionals for guidance.

Managing Intake Of Fiber

By supporting cardiovascular health, moderating blood sugar levels, and encouraging regular bowel movements, dietary fiber significantly contributes to digestive health. In contrast, fiber management necessitates meticulous deliberation for individuals who have an ileostomy to avert potential complications including obstructions, overabundance of flatulence, or diarrhea. Here are some suggestions for managing fiber intake effectively while having an ileostomy:

1. It is crucial to incorporate fiber-rich foods into the diet progressively following ileostomy surgery to provide the digestive system with an opportunity to readjust. Commence by consuming low-fiber alternatives like white rice, white bread, and peeled fruits and vegetables. Gradually introduce higher-fiber foods into your diet as your tolerance improves.

2. Opt for Soluble Fiber: By dissolving in water, soluble fiber creates a gel-like consistency within the digestive tract, facilitating bowel movement regulation without inducing irritation or obstruction. Oatmeal, barley, psyllium husk, as well as specific fruits and vegetables such as apples, carrots, and sweet potatoes, are all excellent sources of soluble fiber.

3. Restrict Insoluble Fiber: Individuals with an ileostomy may find it more difficult to tolerate insoluble fiber, which is present in fresh fruits and

vegetables, whole cereals, nuts, and seeds, due to its relatively unaltered passage through the digestive tract. Although insoluble fiber is essential for overall health, to prevent digestive issues, it may be necessary to limit its intake or ingest it in smaller quantities.

4. It is especially important for individuals with an ileostomy to maintain adequate hydration when consuming foods high in fiber. As fiber facilitates water absorption in the digestive tract, it may increase the risk of dehydration in the event of inadequate fluid intake but may prevent constipation. Ensure that you consume an adequate amount of fluids daily to aid in the elimination and digestion of fiber.

5. Observe Symptoms: Observe how your body reacts to various fiber types and quantities. Manifestations including abdominal pain, bloating, discomfort, or alterations in stool consistency could potentially serve as indicators that dietary modifications or fiber supplementation are

necessary. Keeping a food journal can assist in the identification of discomfort patterns and trigger foods.

6. Fiber supplements may be advantageous for ileostomy patients in certain circumstances, as they aid in the regulation of bowel movements and the promotion of digestive health. Nevertheless, it is imperative to seek the advice of a healthcare professional before incorporating supplements into your routine, given the potential for drug interactions and exacerbation of preexisting digestive conditions.

7. Consult Advisors: Consult a registered dietitian or nutritionist who specializes in gastrointestinal health if you are uncertain about which foods are safe to consume or how to manage your fiber intake while having an ileostomy. They are capable of offering tailored recommendations and assistance to assist you in optimizing your diet and efficiently managing digestive symptoms.

By adhering to these recommendations and collaborating closely with healthcare practitioners, individuals who have an ileostomy can effectively manage their fiber consumption to promote digestive health, and overall well-being, and mitigate the likelihood of complications.

CHAPTER FOUR

Navigating Digestive Obstacles

The possession of an ileostomy can pose distinct difficulties, specifically regarding dietary decisions and adapting to alterations in the digestive system. An ileostomy is a procedure in which the ileum, the lower portion of the small intestine, is obstructed through an abdominal incision, producing a stoma. Managing digestive challenges associated with having an ileostomy frequently necessitates adjusting to novel dietary patterns and comprehending the potential effects of various foods on digestion and stoma functionality.

Comprehending Digestive Alterations:

Individuals who undertake ileostomy surgery may encounter notable alterations in their digestive process. By bypassing the colon, which is responsible for the normal absorption of water and electrolytes, the stoma facilitates an elevation in fluid output. Consequently, electrolyte balance and hydration maintenance become critical. Additionally, the frequency and consistency of bowel movements may be altered by specific foods, which may result in complications like diarrhea or obstructions.

The following are dietary recommendations:

Embracing an ileostomy diet necessitates conscientious decision-making to enhance digestive well-being and comfort. The following are some broad dietary suggestions:

1. It is of the utmost importance that individuals with an ileostomy remain hydrated. Dehydration can be avoided by consuming an adequate amount of fluids, such as water, electrolyte solutions, and hydrating foods like fruits and vegetables.

2. Fiber Consumption: Although fiber is vital for maintaining digestive health, individuals who have an ileostomy may wish to restrict their fiber intake to prevent obstruction. This is because an excessive amount of fiber can result in increased stool output. Choosing sources of soluble fiber such as cooked

vegetables, oatmeal, and bananas may be easier on the digestive system.

3. Restricting the consumption of high-residue foods, including nuts, seeds, raw vegetables, and difficult proteins, can aid in digestion facilitation and mitigate the likelihood of intestinal blockages.

4. Eating smaller, more frequent meals can assist in the management of digestion and the prevention of discomfort that is commonly associated with consuming large meals.

5. Food Trigger Monitoring: Certain foods, including those high in caffeine, piquant substances, or carbonated beverages, may cause digestive symptoms or irritation in the vicinity of the stoma in some individuals. A food journal can assist in the identification and avoidance of potential trigger foods.

Seeking Assistance:

Having an ileostomy-related digestive challenge can place significant emotional and physical strain on the patient. Healthcare professionals, support groups, and online communities can offer invaluable guidance, reassurance, and practical advice regarding ileostomy-related dietary concerns and day-to-day navigating.

Portion Control And Meal Planning

Incorporating meal planning and portion control into the management of an ileostomy diet is crucial for optimal results. Efficient portion control and conscientious meal preparation can contribute to the maintenance of overall health and well-being, reduction of digestive distress, and regulation of digestion in individuals with an ileostomy.

The Significance Of Meal Planning:

By developing a judicious dietary plan, individuals who have an ileostomy can maintain sufficient nutrition despite the difficulties they face with digestion. Consider the subsequent meal planning strategies to be effective:

1. Balanced Nutrition: Strive to include in each meal a selection of nutrient-dense foods, such as fruits, vegetables, lean proteins, complex carbohydrates, and healthy lipids. Give precedence to foods that are digestive system delicate and readily digestible.

2. Maintain Meals Interesting and Pleasurable: Incorporate a variety of food options and recipes into your meal plans. Incorporate a wide range of culinary techniques, flavor profiles, and cultural specialties into your diet to increase variety while maintaining dietary restrictions.

3. Implementing a meal schedule that includes consistent meal times and adequate space between meals can aid in digestion regulation and mitigate the risk of excess. Consume appetizers as necessary and three main meals to sustain energy levels and induce feelings of fullness.

It is critical to monitor portion sizes in individuals who have an ileostomy to minimize digestive symptoms, prevent discomfort, and optimize nutrient absorption. Consider the following portion control suggestions:

1. Engaging in mindful eating practices entails attending to bodily signals of hunger and satiety, savoring each mouthful, and swallowing methodically. It is advisable to refrain from hurrying through meals, as doing so may result in excess and digestive distress.

2. Plate Composition: Aim to achieve a harmonious blend of protein, carbohydrates, and vegetables, paying careful attention to portion sizes. A portion control system may be aided by visual signals, such as the division of platters into sections for various food categories or the use of smaller plates.

3. Food portioning requires the use of measuring containers, utensils, or food scales for precision,

particularly when preparing recipes or serving meals. By doing so, one can effectively manage their caloric intake and guarantee the consumption of suitable portions from every food group.

4. Storage and Departures: To ensure ready-to-eat options, plan meals and divide leftovers into individual containers. This discourages overeating and encourages the practice of portion control at meals and snacking.

Through the implementation of mindful eating, portion control, and balanced nutrition, individuals who have an ileostomy can efficiently regulate their dietary intake, foster optimal digestive health, and augment their overall state of being.

Particular Considerations For Children Having An Ileostomy

Children who have an ileostomy encounter distinct obstacles when it comes to dietary management and adjusting to life with a prosthetic device. Irrespective of the duration of the ileostomy, parental and caregiver involvement is vital in ensuring that the infant receives adequate nutrition and fosters sound development.

Nutrition Appropriate For Age:

It is critical to provide age-appropriate sustenance to children who have an ileostomy to ensure their optimal physical and cognitive development is supported. Dietary considerations for adolescents with an ileostomy include the following:

1. Offer an assortment of nutrient-dense foods to satisfy your child's nutritional requirements, such as fruits, vegetables, whole cereals, lean proteins, and dairy products. Promote the exploration of diverse flavors and sensations to broaden individuals' palates and foster a more varied diet.

2. Maintain vigilance over your child's fluid consumption to avert dehydration, especially in instances of high temperature or physical exertion.

The provision of electrolyte solutions, water, and hydrating foods such as cucumber and cantaloupe is essential for maintaining adequate hydration.

3. Implement a gradual introduction of foods rich in fiber and closely monitor your child's tolerance to such foods to mitigate the risk of digestive discomfort or complications, including blockages. To promote digestive health, choose soluble fiber sources such as applesauce, pureed bananas, and well-cooked vegetables.

4. Specialized Formulas: A healthcare provider may prescribe specialized formulas or nutritional supplements for children with particular dietary restrictions or nutritional requirements, which may prove advantageous in certain instances.

Collaborate diligently with the healthcare team responsible for your child to guarantee that all of their nutritional needs are satiated.

Ensuring a nurturing mealtime atmosphere and imparting knowledge regarding their condition can foster a sense of empowerment and self-assurance in children with an ileostomy regarding the management of their dietary requirements. Take into consideration the subsequent approaches:

1. Foster an environment that promotes candid dialogue with your child regarding their ileostomy, elucidating its purpose and the physiological ramifications it may have on their digestive system. Employ language that is suitable for their age and offers reassurance and assistance as they confront their dietary preferences and obstacles.

2. Active Participation in Meal Preparation: Encourage your child to develop a positive attitude towards food and foster independence by engaging in meal preparation activities, including grocery shopping, cooking, and meal planning. Permit them to select their preferred cuisines and engage in the process of determining meal options.

3. Peer support and education: Establish connections with other families and participate in support organizations catering to children with ileostomies to exchange insights, counsel, and offer emotional solace. Promoting social interaction among children who may be experiencing comparable obstacles can cultivate a sense of community and belonging.

4. Consistent Follow-Up Care: It is advisable to arrange periodic follow-up appointments with the healthcare team to monitor your child's progress, nutritional requirements, and stoma functionality. Ensure that any inquiries or concerns about their digestion, diet, or general health are addressed throughout these appointments.

Parents and caregivers can facilitate the well-being and satisfaction of children with an ileostomy by implementing the following strategies: ensuring proper nutrition, encouraging candid dialogue, and providing diligent care.

CHAPTER FIVE

Diet For Ileostomy During Pregnancy

To ensure optimal maternal and fetal health, managing an ileostomy diet during pregnancy requires meticulous planning, monitoring, and collaboration with healthcare providers. Pregnancy can present individuals with an ileostomy with distinct challenges and factors to be mindful of, encompassing alterations in dietary requirements, metabolic functionality, and stoma maintenance.

Nutritional Factors To Consider:

Pregnancy induces heightened physiological demands, which require mothers and fetuses to modify their dietary habits to promote optimal health. The following nutritional considerations should be taken into account by pregnant women with ileostomies:

1. It is important to monitor caloric intake during pregnancy to maintain sufficient energy levels and promote healthy weight gain. Prioritize the

consumption of nutrient-dense foods that are rich in essential vitamins, minerals, and macronutrients to adequately meet the heightened nutritional requirements during pregnancy.

2. It is advisable to seek guidance from a healthcare professional regarding the necessity of prenatal vitamins or particular nutrient supplements to prevent deficiencies and promote the growth and progress of both the mother and the fetus. During pregnancy, iron, folic acid, calcium, and vitamin D are among the most important nutrients to consider.

3. Hydration: Sustain adequate fluid intake throughout the day by consuming a variety of hydrating foods and beverages, including water, herbal infusions, and fruits and vegetables. During pregnancy, dehydration can both worsen digestive symptoms and elevate the likelihood of developing complications.

4. A Diet Rich in Fiber: To prevent constipation, a prevalent issue during pregnancy, integrate foods

abundant in fiber into your intake. This will facilitate regular digestive movements. Adjust your intake accordingly, bearing in mind that high-fiber foods may exacerbate digestive issues or stoma output.

Sustaining And Observing Stoma:

The functioning of a stoma may be impacted by pregnancy, which may require modifications to stoma care regimens and appliance administration. Vigilantly observe the appearance of the stoma, the consistency of the outflow, and the integrity of the epidermis. Immediately seek medical attention if any indications of complications or concerns arise.

1. Appliance Selection: Opt for stoma appliances that fit the evolving dimensions and contours of the stoma throughout pregnancy, while also offering sufficient support and security. It is advisable to seek guidance from a stoma care nurse or healthcare provider to ensure appropriate fit and compatibility with one's evolving body.

2. Prevent irritation, moisture accumulation, and friction on the peristomal epidermis by employing barrier lotions, protective powders, and suitable ostomy accessories. Maintain proper skin hygiene and inspect the area surrounding the stoma frequently for indications of irritation or deterioration.

3. Stoma Prolapse or Retraction: Changes in abdominal pressure and muscle tone associated with pregnancy may elevate the likelihood of stoma prolapse or retraction. Observe the appearance and function of the stoma and notify your healthcare provider of any concerns or changes for evaluation and management.

Collaborative Support And Care:

It is imperative to uphold transparent lines of communication with healthcare professionals, such as dietitians, obstetricians, and stoma care nurses, to ensure comprehensive care and address any concerns that may arise during pregnancy. Be proactive in communicating your specific dietary, stoma care, and pregnancy management requirements, concerns, and preferences.

1. Prenatal Counseling: It is advisable to consult healthcare professionals who possess expertise in the administration of ileostomies during pregnancy for prenatal counseling and guidance. Analyze potential hazards, obstacles, and approaches to achieving optimal outcomes for both the mother and the fetus while juggling the responsibilities of an ileostomy.

2. Support Network: Throughout your pregnancy, rely on your support network of family, friends, and fellow ostomates for emotional solace, practical guidance, and the exchange of personal experiences. Establish connections with advocacy organizations, online communities, and support groups to gain access to additional resources and encouragement.

3. To foster both physical and emotional well-being throughout pregnancy, it is imperative to give precedence to self-care practices, stress management techniques, and relaxation strategies. During

pregnancy and stoma maintenance, it is important to pay attention to one's body, take necessary leisure, and participate in enjoyable and satisfying activities.

Ileostomy patients can successfully navigate pregnancy by adopting a collaborative care approach, advocating for their specific requirements, and placing self-care and well-being as top priorities. This will inspire confidence and resilience in the patient.

In summary, the management of an ileostomy diet necessitates the ability to navigate dietary obstacles, adjust to fluctuations in digestion, and place nutritional requirements and general health as top priorities. Individuals who have an ileostomy can improve their quality of life, and optimize digestive health, and accomplish this by adopting mindful feeding practices, seeking guidance from healthcare professionals, and cultivating a positive relationship with food.

Having an ileostomy can necessitate substantial lifestyle adjustments, including modifications to one's diet. Although dining out with an ileostomy may appear intimidating at first, it can be transformed into a pleasurable experience with adequate planning and consciousness.

1. Preparing Ahead:

It is advisable to conduct a prior investigation on restaurants that offer a varied menu that includes options that are suitable for individuals who have ileostomies. Presently, a multitude of dining establishments provides lighter and healthier supper options, which may be more accommodating to the digestive system.

2. Decision-Making Caution:

Choose foods that are readily digestible to reduce the likelihood of discomfort or obstruction. In terms of overall safety, steamed vegetables, grilled proteins, and well-cooked cereals are preferable alternatives. Potential health problems can be avoided by avoiding high-fiber foods, including difficult meats and uncooked vegetables.

3. Remain Hydrated:

It is critical to maintain sufficient hydration, particularly for those who have an ileostomy. Water or other non-caffeinated beverages should be chosen to maintain hydration levels while dining out. Alcohol and caffeine restriction can additionally aid in the prevention of electrolyte imbalances and dehydration.

4. Control of Portion:

A portion control system should be utilized to prevent excess, which can cause unwarranted stress on the digestive system. It is advisable to contemplate ordering smaller portions or sharing meals with dining companions as strategies to mitigate discomfort and enhance digestion.

5. Prepare yourself:

Carry essential items, including additional ostomy bags and tissues, for use in the event of an emergency. Obtain prior knowledge of the locations of restrooms so that you can quickly access them if necessary.

6. Interact with Staff:

Please feel at liberty to communicate your dietary requirements and restrictions to the restaurant personnel. They are frequently flexible and can assist in tailoring dishes to meet specific dietary needs. Additionally, requesting condiments and garnishes on the side can aid in ingredient portion control.

7. Observe your body: Observe how your body reacts to various substances and environments. One may contemplate future avoidance of specific dishes that consistently elicit distress or symptoms.

8. Delight in the Experience:

Notwithstanding dietary adjustments, dining out ought to continue to be a pleasurable and communal experience. Savor the company of loved ones and friends while attending to the requirements of your body and appreciating the culinary experience.

CHAPTER SIX

The Psychological And Emotional Consequences Of Dietary Alterations

Eating and dietary modifications necessitated by an ileostomy can elicit a variety of psychological and emotional reactions.

Pupils may undergo emotional responses ranging from sorrow to frustration in response to the perceived disruption of their usual routines. It is critical to confront these emotions to cultivate acceptance and advance one's general state of well-being.

1. Adaptation and Acceptance:

Recognize and embrace the dietary modifications as an essential component of living with an ileostomy. Recognize that while transitioning to a modified diet may require some perseverance and time, it in no way compromises an individual's standard of living.

2. Request Support:

Establish connections with support groups or consult healthcare professionals who possess expertise in ostomy care for guidance. Validation and reassurance can be obtained by sharing one's experiences with others who have been through similar obstacles.

3. Preserve Perspective:

Concentrate on the benefits of dietary modifications, including enhanced health outcomes and symptom management. Embrace novel gastronomic experiences and investigate alternative preparation techniques and ingredients.

4. Engage in Self-Compassion:

When experiencing disappointment or frustration, be kind to yourself. It is important to recognize that making dietary adjustments is a continuous process, and experiencing setbacks is an expected aspect of the journey.

5. Develop Your Resilience:

Formulate adaptive mechanisms to manage the emotional peaks and valleys that accompany modifications to one's diet. Participate in stress-relieving and relaxation-promoting activities, such as engaging in meditative meditation or pursuing creative expression.

6. Communication Openness:

Discuss candidly with close friends and family the emotional repercussions of dietary modifications. The act of voicing anxieties and concerns has the potential to cultivate empathy and fortify interpersonal connections.

7. Commemorate Advances:

Regardless of their size, acknowledge and commemorate milestones along the dietary voyage. Every incremental progress made in the direction of acceptance and adaptation is a noteworthy accomplishment that merits recognition.

8. Professional Assistance:

One should contemplate enrolling in professional counseling or therapy to confront latent emotional difficulties and cultivate adaptive coping strategies. A mental health professional is capable of providing individualized guidance and assistance that is specifically designed to address one's unique requirements.

Soliciting Expert Dietary Guidance

To effectively manage dietary modifications after ileostomy, it is imperative to seek the counsel of healthcare experts who possess specialized knowledge in ostomy care and nutrition.

By consulting with a qualified dietitian, individuals can enhance their nutritional consumption, alleviate symptoms, and enhance their general state of health.

1. A consultation at the dietary consultant level:

Make arrangements to meet with a registered dietitian who possesses expertise in providing care for patients with ileostomies. In addition to evaluating nutritional requirements, a dietitian can offer individualized dietary suggestions and attend to particular issues concerning digestion and absorption.

2. Tailored Meal Preparation:

Consult a dietitian to formulate a personalized meal strategy that reflects specific dietary restrictions, personal preferences, and health objectives. Promoting gastrointestinal health and preventing nutrient deficiencies are two benefits of a well-balanced diet.

3. Monitoring and Modification:

Consistently assess dietary consumption and symptoms, and consult a dietitian for guidance on any required modifications. Meal plans that are modified by an individual's food reaction can be optimized for digestion and discomfort reduction.

4. Provision of Resources and Education:

Leverage educational resources offered by healthcare professionals, such as support groups, informational materials, and cuisine demonstrations. The provision of knowledge and skills to individuals fosters self-management and instills confidence in the selection of dietary options.

5. Affiliation with Lifestyle Elements:

Other variables besides dietary consumption that could potentially influence digestion and general health include stress management, physical activity, and hydration. By adopting a holistic strategy towards modifying one's lifestyle, substantial enhancements in gastrointestinal health are possible.

6. Care Collaboration:

Encourage collaborative efforts and transparent dialogue among healthcare professionals engaged in ostomy care, such as dietitians, surgeons, and nurses.

A multidisciplinary approach guarantees comprehensive assistance and synchronized oversight of dietary and medical requirements.

7. Compliance and Adherence:

Promoting compliance with dietary recommendations and treatment plans can be achieved using continuous education, positive reinforcement, and encouragement.

Effectively addressing obstacles to adherence and offering pragmatic approaches can significantly augment sustained achievement.

8. Long-Term Assistance:

Acknowledge the significance of ongoing support and follow-up care after the preliminary phases of dietary modification. Consistent consultations with healthcare professionals facilitate continuous assessment of nutritional status, management of symptoms, and modification of dietary interventions as required.

In summary, successfully managing dietary modifications while having an ileostomy necessitates a comprehensive strategy that incorporates pragmatic approaches, psychological assistance, and expert advice. By adopting a proactive approach and cultivating resilience, individuals can accept dietary modifications as an integral component of a gratifying and self-assured way of life.

CHAPTER SEVEN

Tailored Ileostomy Dietary Strategies

Through the creation of an orifice in the abdominal wall called an ileostomy, the ileum, the distal portion of the small intestine, is elevated to the skin's surface. Using this aperture, referred to as a stoma, bodily waste is expelled into an external receptacle. In many cases, individuals who have undergone ileostomy must modify their dietary patterns to account for alterations in nutrient absorption and assimilation. To promote overall health and well-being, ensure adequate nutrition, and manage symptoms, individualized ileostomy diet plans are vital.

The fundamental tenet of a personalized ileostomy diet plan is to accommodate the unique requirements and inclinations of every individual by customizing dietary selections. Due to the substantial impact that the removal of the large intestine has on metabolism and assimilation, it may be imperative to make specific dietary adjustments to avert complications including malnutrition, electrolyte imbalances, and dehydration.

When formulating an individualized ileostomy diet plan, it is critical to prioritize foods that are digestively simple and have a low propensity to induce obstruction or irritation in the vicinity of the stoma. It is common to advise consuming low-fiber foods, including thoroughly cooked vegetables, lean meats, white bread, and refined cereals, to reduce the likelihood of intestinal obstruction and associated discomfort.

Ileostomy patients must also be mindful of their fluid consumption, in addition to making informed decisions regarding the selection of suitable foods. Maintaining adequate hydration is of utmost importance as dehydration and electrolyte imbalances may result from increased fluid loss through the stoma. Oral rehydration solutions, electrolyte-rich beverages, copious amounts of water, and clear stews can assist in preserving fluid balance and averting complications.

In addition, it is critical to provide sufficient amounts of protein, vitamins, and minerals in one's diet to facilitate immune function, promote overall health, and support tissue repair. In the aftermath of surgery, lean meats, fish, poultry, eggs, dairy products, and fortified foods may supply vital nutrients required for recovery and restoration.

To formulate an individualized ileostomy diet plan, it is imperative to seek guidance from a healthcare professional, such as a registered dietitian, given the substantial variation in dietary requirements among individuals. Dietitians possess the ability to evaluate the nutritional needs of individuals, attend to particular apprehensions or dietary limitations, and offer pragmatic advice regarding meal preparation, food selection, and portion control.

In essence, individualized ileostomy diet plans are crucial in fostering the highest level of health and wellness among ileostomy-dependent individuals. Enhancing nutrient intake, maintaining proper hydration, and prioritizing easily digestible foods are all strategies that can aid in the prevention of complications, promote healing, and enhance overall quality of life.

Frequent Difficulties And Solutions

The presence of an ileostomy creates distinct obstacles that may have repercussions on one's dietary patterns, nutritional standing, and overall standard of living. To effectively manage an ileostomy and sustain a healthy lifestyle, it is critical to comprehend and confront these challenges.

A prevalent obstacle encountered by individuals who have an ileostomy is the potential for dehydration and electrolyte imbalances as a result of heightened fluid loss via the stoma. Especially during periods of high output or in humid weather, this may occur. Consistently consuming a sufficient amount of fluids throughout the day is crucial for preventing dehydration. Additionally, oral rehydration solutions and electrolyte-rich beverages can aid in restoring electrolyte balance and preventing complications.

An additional obstacle pertains to the potential for intestinal obstructions or blockages to arise, a consequence of undigested food or fibrous substances becoming ensnared within the digestive tract. It is frequently recommended that individuals adhere to a low-fiber diet and refrain from consuming fibrous meats, raw vegetables, nuts, and seeds, to mitigate this risk. Additionally, consuming small, frequent meals and chewing food thoroughly can aid in the prevention of blockages and facilitate digestion.

In addition, skin irritation or discomfort may be experienced by some individuals in the vicinity of the stoma as a result of adhesive allergies, friction, or discharge.

Adequate ostomy care, which consists of routine cleansing, application of suitable skin barriers, and choice of ostomy products, can aid in the prevention of skin complications and the promotion of healing. Seeking the counsel of an ostomy nurse or healthcare provider regarding stoma care techniques and product selection can yield invaluable insights.

Additionally, numerous individuals may find it difficult to adapt to the psychological and emotional facets of ileostomy life.

It is not uncommon to experience anxiety, depression, or feelings of self-consciousness as a result of enduring such a substantial surgical procedure. Engaging in support group participation, counseling, or establishing connections with like-minded individuals can provide significant emotional solace, motivation, and pragmatic coping mechanisms.

In essence, effectively managing the typical difficulties that arise from having an ileostomy necessitates the implementation of pragmatic approaches, psychological assistance, and proactive personal hygiene.

Individuals can successfully tolerate and maintain a healthy ileostomy by remaining well-informed, requesting professional advice, and establishing connections with support networks.

Sustained Adherence To A Healthful Ileostomy Diet

For those who have an ileostomy to preserve their long-term health and quality of life, a nutritious diet is vital. Although there may be dietary modifications and restrictions in place during the immediate post-operative phase, the ultimate objective is to develop enduring eating patterns that nurture overall well-being, avert complications, and facilitate efficient assimilation and absorption of nutrients.

The maintenance of a healthy ileostomy diet over the long term requires an emphasis on variety and balance. By incorporating a variety of nutrient-dense foods into one's diet, such as fruits, vegetables, whole cereals, lean proteins, and healthy lipids, one can promote overall health and guarantee sufficient consumption of vital nutrients.

By experimenting with new recipes, culinary techniques, and food combinations, one can enhance the appeal and enjoyment of meals.

Consistently monitoring stoma output and modifying dietary decisions in response is an additional critical element of long-term dietary management. Monitoring the consistency, frequency, and volume of bowel movements can yield significant insights regarding the impact of various foods and beverages on digestion and elimination. By making modifications to portion sizes, adjusting fiber intake, and avoiding potential trigger foods, individuals can mitigate digestive symptoms and enhance their overall comfort and well-being.

Consistent monitoring of nutritional status and hydration levels is imperative for the preservation of long-term health, in conjunction with dietary considerations. Regular evaluation of nutrient concentrations, including electrolytes, vitamins, and minerals, can facilitate the detection of imbalances or deficiencies that may necessitate dietary modifications or supplementation. It is imperative to maintain adequate hydration throughout the day to support optimal stoma function and prevent dehydration.

Furthermore, the integration of healthful lifestyle practices, including consistent engagement in physical activity, effective management of stress, sufficient sleep, and abstinence from tobacco use, can significantly augment both general welfare and gastrointestinal functionality. Consistent physical activity has been shown to enhance digestion, facilitate regular bowel movements, elevate mood, and increase energy. Aside from improving overall quality of life, stress management techniques such as mindfulness, relaxation exercises, and hobbies can aid in the reduction of digestive symptoms associated with stress.

In conclusion, maintaining knowledge and taking an active role in addressing concerns regarding stoma care, dietary recommendations, and self-management techniques are critical for ensuring sustained success and self-assurance in the management of an ileostomy. Obtaining continuous support from healthcare professionals, ostomy nurses, dietitians, and support groups can furnish one with invaluable encouragement, practical advice, and resources to help one navigate the complexities and advantages of ileostomy life.

In summary, sustained adherence to a nutritious ileostomy diet necessitates a variety of practices, including mindful eating, balanced nutrition, effective hydration management, lifestyle adjustments, and proactive self-care. Through the adoption of a holistic approach to health and wellness, education, and nutrition, individuals with an ileostomy can enhance their digestive health, avert complications, and sustain a physically active and satisfying way of life.

Conclusion

In summary, the ileostomy diet is of paramount importance in preserving the health and overall well-being of individuals who have undergone ileostomy surgery. The primary objectives of this dietary plan are symptom relief, avertience of complications, and enhancement of general health. During this process of dietary adjustment, individuals gain the ability to acclimate to their altered digestive system by selecting foods that are well-informed, maximize the absorption of nutrients, and minimize any potential discomfort.

Adhering to a diet low in fiber to mitigate the likelihood of intestinal blockages, maintaining adequate hydration to prevent dehydration and electrolyte imbalances, and progressively reintroducing specific foods to assess tolerance levels are the fundamental tenets of an ileostomy diet. Although it may appear restrictive at first glance, the ileostomy diet provides an extensive array of nourishing choices, such as cooked vegetables, fruits without seeds and skins, lean proteins, and refined grains.

Furthermore, it is critical to uphold a well-rounded dietary regimen that is abundant in vital nutrients, vitamins, and fluids to sustain optimal energy levels and promote overall well-being. Collaboration between individuals undergoing ileostomy and healthcare professionals, including dietitians, is of the utmost importance to tailor their dietary regimen to their particular requirements and inclinations.

In conclusion, individuals who adhere to a meticulously designed ileostomy diet and practice mindful eating can effectively cope with their condition, optimize digestive functionality, and reestablish a gratifying way of life following surgery.

THE END

9 798880 169863